Diabetes Solution: Diabetes Guide On How To Incorporate Diabetes Diet And Nutrition Plan For A Diabetes Free Lifestyle

Introduction

I want to thank you and congratulate you for downloading the book, *"Diabetes Solution: Diabetes Guide on How to Incorporate Diabetes Diet and Nutrition Plan for a Diabetes Free Lifestyle"*.

This book contains proven steps and strategies on how to incorporate diabetes cooking strategies into actual day-to-day meal plans.

What is diabetes? What are the recommended foods in a diabetes diet? What are the foods to avoid? How do you create your own meal plan? What are the different approaches to a diabetes diet? What are the different easy-to-cook recipes that could be included in the Diabetes meal plan? These questions will be answered in this book.

Thanks again for downloading this book, I hope you enjoy it!

Chapter 1: Introducing the Diabetes Meal Plan

What is Diabetes?

Diabetes mellitus or more commonly known as Diabetes is a metabolic disease in which the patient has high blood sugar, either because the body does not respond to insulin or insulin production is insufficient. It is characterized by symptoms such as excessive thirst and increased frequency of urination, weight loss, and fatigue, lack of interest, tiredness, excessive hunger, and blurred vision.

Whatever you choose to eat, every meal makes a great deal of difference in your blood pressure, blood glucose and cholesterol. Eating healthy foods shouldn't be difficult! You just have to be properly guided with a great meal plan.

A meal plan is a scientifically determined guide that helps you determine the right kind and amount of food that you should eat. An ideal meal plan for diabetes should take into consideration the following: the plate method, glycemic index, and carb counting. Medical Nutrition Therapy, more commonly known as the Diabetes diet, is simply a healthy-living meal plan characterized by foods that are low in fat and calories but rich in nutrients, with emphasis on whole grains, veggies and fruits. Contrary to what most people think, the Diabetes diet is not a restrictive diet. In fact, it is the ideal diet plan for almost everybody! It will help you slowly improve your blood pressure, blood glucose and cholesterol. What makes the diabetes meal plan special is that you not only prevent and control your diabetes but it also helps you lose weight!

Recommended Foods

A diabetes meal plan is typically composed of the following:

- Fiber – What makes fiber essential for a Diabetes diet is that it normalizes digestion and bowel movement, aides in losing weight, prevents colorectal cancer, decreases the body's cholesterol levels, and helps control and decrease the body's blood sugar levels. According to the research conducted by experts from the Institute of Medicine in 2012, young women (younger than 50) should take 25 grams of fiber while men should take 38 grams every day. Foods like oats, nuts, citrus fruits, green beans, peas, potatoes, carrots, beans, wheat bran, potatoes, cauliflower, barley, apples, psyllium, and whole-wheat flour are examples of fiber-rich foods.

- Healthy Carbohydrates – What are the good carbs? Over the last few years, carbohydrates have become the sworn enemy of women. Carbohydrates are both avoided and feared. But carbohydrates are a vital part of our diet because they give us the energy that we need in order to accomplish our day-to-day tasks. The trick is to select healthy sources of carbs. A diet rich in healthy carbs could reduce one's chances of having diabetes, coronary artery disease, and cancer. Foods that are rich in healthy carbohydrates are the following: beans, nuts, low-fat dairy foods, unprocessed foods, whole grains, fruits and vegetables.

- Good Fats – These are foods which contain polyunsaturated and monounsaturated fats, such as avocados, pecans, almonds, canola, olive, walnuts and peanut oils. Good fats can help you decrease your cholesterol levels. However, they should be eaten sparingly since they are also high in calories.

- Fish – Make sure that you include heart-healthy fish in your weekly diet. Fish could be an alternative to meats because they have relatively lower amounts of fats. For example, fishes like tuna, halibut and cod contain lower amounts of saturated fat, total fat, and cholesterol compared to meat and poultry. Fish varieties such as bluefish, tuna, mackerel and salmon contain high amounts of omega-3 fatty acids which aid in promoting heart health by lowering triglycerides in the blood. However, as much as possible, avoid fishes like swordfish, king mackerel and tile fish because they contain high levels of mercury.

Foods to Avoid

Foods which contain the following could go against your goal of preventing or controlling diabetes and increase your risk of stroke and heart disease by accelerating the growth of hardened and clogged arteries.

- Saturated fats – These include foods that contain high-fat animal proteins, such as hot dogs, bacon, sausage, beef, and daily products. As much as possible, completely eliminate them from your diet or at least get no more than 5% of your daily calorie intake from saturated fats.

- Cholesterol – Examples of foods that are high in cholesterol are the following: egg yolks, proteins, liver, shellfish and other organ meats. Make sure that you aim for less than 300 mg of cholesterol-derived calories every day.

- Sodium – Make sure that you take less than 2,300 mg of Sodium every day. Foods that contain high amounts of sodium are the following: table salt, baking powder, baking soda, soy sauce, salad dressings, sauces, cooked bacon, cheese, cucumber pickles and cheese.

- Transfats – These are fats that can be found in processed foods, baked goods, and margarines. They should be completely eliminated from one's diet.

Putting Everything Together

The following are the most common approaches in creating an optimized diabetes diet that seeks to keep your blood glucose within the healthy range. You have to remember that they are subjective. What might work for John might not work for Peter. You have to consult your physician or dietitian to find an approach (or combination of approaches) that would easily fit your lifestyle.

- Counting "Carbs" Technique - One of the primary roles of insulin is to break down glucose molecules. Therefore, they play a major role in controlling the blood glucose level. You have to make sure that the amount and timing of carbohydrates is constant each day, especially if you take insulin or other diabetes medications. Otherwise, your blood sugar level might fluctuate more often. Counting carbs works by measuring proportions of food, reading food levels, and paying attention to counting your carbohydrate intake in each meal.

- The exchange system works by first grouping the foods into primary categories: meats, carbohydrates, fats and meat substitutes. One serving of each category is called "exchange." An exchange of the same amount (of protein, fat, carbohydrates and calories) has the same effect on blood sugar. For example, you can trade one exchange of apple for 1/3 cup of white pasta when it comes to your carbohydrate intake.

- Dietitians normally recommend the usage of the Glycemic index when selecting carbohydrates. Unlike those with low Glycemic index, foods with high GI significantly increase blood sugar levels. Foods like brown bread, cereals, whole-grain oats, and brown rice have a lower Glycemic index compared to highly processed foods like white rice and white bread.

Sample Meal Plan

Your meal plan should take into consideration your weight and your physical activity level. The following menu is created for someone who needs to consume 1,200 – 1,600 calories every day.

Day 1

For breakfast, you will have whole-wheat waffles, six ounces of non fat yogurt and ¾ cup of fresh berries. For lunch, you will have a medium-sized apple, a tablespoon of almond butter, and cheese and veggie pita. For dinner, you will have salad composed of the following: 2 cups of spinach, ¼ cup of chopped bell pepper, 2 teaspoons of red wine vinegar, ½ tomato and 2 teaspoons of olive oil. For snacks, you will have 2 pieces of unsalted rice cakes with non-fat cheese and a piece of medium-sized orange.

Day 2

For breakfast, you will have 2 slices of whole wheat toast, 1 teaspoon of margarine, 8 ounces of skimmed milk, ½ grapefruit and 1 poached egg. For your morning snack, you will have six ounces of vanilla-flavored nonfat yogurt. For lunch, you will have 2 slices of whole wheat bread, 2 ounces of sliced turkey, 1 tablespoon of light mayonnaise, ¾ cup of pineapple, 1 cup of tomato and cucumber salad, and 2 tablespoons of nonfat Italian Dressing. For your afternoon snack, you will have a cup of cubed cantaloupe, 1 piece of sliced red pepper and 2 tablespoons of ranch dressing. For dinner, you will have 3 ounces of pork loin roast, ½ pear, 1 cup of roasted potato, and 1 cup of steamed asparagus. For your midnight snack, you will have 5 ounces of light yogurt, 1 tablespoon of peanut butter, 7 ounces of skimmed milk and 1 toasted waffle (low fat).

Day 3

For breakfast, you will have one serving of vanilla-flavored Up 'n Go instant breakfast, a piece of toasted brown bread, and tea with low-fat milk. For your morning snack, you will have 25g apple and raisin cake and coffee with low-fat milk. For lunch, you will have 50 g grilled chicken breast (skinned), ½ cup of baked beans in tomato sauce, 120g peeled orange, lettuce and cucumber salad, and tea with low-fat milk. For your afternoon snack, you will have 25g of dark fruitcake and tea with low fat milk. For supper, you will have 50g lean pork chop, 40g sliced pineapple, ½ cup of steamed broccoli, ¼ cup of carrot salad, a slice of brown bread and tea with low-fat milk.

Day 4

For breakfast, you will have ½ cup of ProNutro, 50g of boiled egg, 1 slice of whole-wheat bread and tea with low-fat milk. For morning snack, you will have 2 biscuits of Pro-Vita multigrain and coffee with low-fat milk. For lunch, you will have a club sandwich made of the following ingredients: 50g lean and sliced roast beef (fat removed), sliced gherkins, tomatoes and lettuce, 90g of sliced papaya, 2 slices of seed loaf, 100 ml low-fat yogurt and tea with low-fat milk.

Day 5

For breakfast, you will have a serving of All-Bran cereal with ½ cup of low-fat milk or plain yoghurt, omega-3 bread (wholegrain) with diabetic jam and tea with 30ml low-fat milk. For morning snack, you will have a small apple and tea with low fat milk. For lunch, you will have 60g banana. ½ cup of fresh cucumber, ½ cup of tinned asparagus, 1 slice of Rye bread with 2 teaspoons of Lite margarine and 50g tuna with 1 teaspoon low-fat salad dressing. For afternoon snack, you will have 15g coffee muffin and tea with low fat milk. For supper, you will have 50g grilled lamb chop, ½ cup of cooked brown rice, watercress and lettuce salad, 18g dried apricots, ½ cup of steamed green beans with 185g of herbs and ½ cup of lemon juice.

Day 6

For breakfast, you will have ½ cup of maze meal porridge with ½ cup of low fat milk, 20g of grilled bacon, a slice of toasted brown bread (seeded) with 2 teaspoons Lite margarine, grilled tomato, and tea with low-fat milk. For morning snack, you will have 2Pro-Vita biscuits with 2 teaspoons of fat-free cottage cheese. For lunch, you will have 50g of Chicken and mushroom casserole, ½ cup of cooked peas, ½ cup of beetroot salad, ½ cup of Basmati rice, 120g of Naartjie segments and tea with low-fat milk. For afternoon snack, you will have 2 pieces of fresh plums and ½ cup of Peartiser. For supper, you will have 50g of grilled Kabeljou with chili, 90g baked potato with 2 tablespoons of herbs and 30g of garlic, ½ cup of cooked spinach, 1 serving of cabbage carrot salad, ½ cup of strawberries, 70ml low fat yogurt and tea with low-fat milk.

Day 7

For breakfast, you will have ½ cup of mixed berry muesli with ½ cup of low-fat milk, 15g grated cheese, 25g date and banana muffin with 1 teaspoon of Lite margarine, and tea with low-fat milk. For morning snack, you will have 15g raisins, 15g of peanuts and tea with low-fat milk. For lunch, you will have 50g grilled lean steal, lettuce, cucumber and tomato salad, 120g pear, 100 ml low fat yogurt and tea with low-fat milk. For your afternoon snack, you will have 50g lean tomato mince, ½ cup of cooked Durum pasta, celery and apple salad with ½ cup of low fat salad dressing, ½ cup of steamed veggies, 100g sliced plums and tea with low-fat milk.

Day 8

For breakfast, you will have one serving of original-flavored Oats-So-Easy with ½ cup of low-fat milk, 50g scrambled egg, a slice of toasted whole-wheat bread, and tea with low fat milk. For morning snack, you will have 33 g of strawberry-flavored fruit bar and tea with low-fat milk. For lunch, you will have 50g grilled Sosaties, 90g baked potato, ½ cup of Spanspek, ½ cup of French bean salad with low-fat dressing, and tea with low-fat milk. For supper, you will have ½ cup of cooked brown rice, ½ cup of aubergine cooked with onions and tomatoes, 120g of sliced orange, ½ cup of gherkin, lettuce and tomato salad, and tea with low-fat milk.

Day 9

For breakfast, you will have ½ cup of cooked Tastee wheat with low-fat milk, 1 serving of poached egg, a slice of brown loaf bread with 2 teaspoons of Lite margarine and tea with low-fat milk. For morning snack, you will have a 110g of fresh grapes and tea with low fat milk. For lunch, you will have 50g grilled lean steak, ½ cup of lightly boiled snap peas, ½ cup of fresh cherries, 1/3 cup of cabbage and carrot salad with low fat, 2 tablespoons of yogurt, pineapple-flavored yogurt, and tea with low-fat milk. For afternoon snack, you will have a slice of banana loaf and tea with low-fat milk. For supper, you will have 50g roasted chicken, ¼ cup of avocado and green pepper salad with low-fat dressing, ½ cup of three-bean salad, 1 cup of mixed berries, and tea with low-fat milk.

Day 10

For breakfast, you will have ¾ cup of plain flake oatmeal topped with ¼ cup of sunflower seeds, a pinch of cinnamon and 2 tablespoons of raisins and a cup of skimmed milk. For lunch, you will have a slice of Pumpernickel open-faced sandwich with 1 teaspoon of mustard, spinach and 60g of roasted turkey. For dinner, you will have spinach salad (composed of a cup of spinach, 1 diced tomato, 1 tablespoon of fat-free salad dressing and 2 tablespoons of shredded carrot) and Red Pepper and Asparagus Omelet (composed of 2 egg whites, 2 tablespoons of water, ½ cup of red pepper and ½ cup of asparagus spear).

Day 11

For breakfast, you will have a cup of high-fiber cereal, ¼ cup of walnuts, 1 medium-sized pear and 250 ml skimmed milk. For lunch, you will have a serving of pita pizza (composed of whole wheat pita, 1 serving of vegetable of your choosing, 1 tablespoon of low sodium tomato sauce, and 2 ounces of partly skimmed mozzarella cheese), 2 medium sized plums, and 250 ml carrot and celery sticks. For dinner, you will have 60g baked salmon, 1 cup of steamed broccoli and cauliflower, 1 medium-sized baked potato and ½ cup of canned peaches.

Day 12

For breakfast, you will have 2 slices of whole grain toast with 2 teaspoon of non-hydrogenated margarine, apple, scrambled eggs (composed of 1 egg, 1/3 cup of skimmed milk, vegetables and low-fat cheddar cheese), and tea with low-fat milk. For lunch, you will have salmon salad with 1 ½ cup of salad greens, ½ cup of sliced red pepper, ½ cup of cherry tomatoes, 2 ounces baked salmon and 1 tablespoon of fat-free salad dressing. For dinner, you will have Stir Fried Sweet Chili Tofu, 1 cup of brown rice and 250ml cantaloupe.

Chapter 2: Diabetes Recipes

The following are some recipes that can be incorporated into your diabetes meal plan:

Stir Fried Sweet Chili Tofu

This dish requires a cooking time of 12 minutes and 15 minutes of preparation time. This recipe yields 4 servings. The following are the ingredients for this dish:

- Vegetable cooking spray

- ½ cup of red bell pepper

- ¾ cup of firm tofu

- ½ cup of vegetable broth

- A cup of sliced Spanish onion

- ¼ cup of sweet chili sauce

- A cup of broccoli florets

- 1 teaspoon of grated orange zest

- 1 cup of baby carrots

- ¾ cup of trimmed sugar snap peas

- 1 teaspoon of chopped fresh cilantro

Instructions:

Heat a medium-sized skillet over medium-high heat. Spray it with the cooking spray. Cook tofu on both sides until brown. Remove from the pan. Set aside. Sauté onion for 1 minute. Toss in the peas, broccoli, red pepper and carrots. Stir-fry until crisp, or for 5 minutes. Return the tofu and add the broth, orange zest and chili sauce. Heat until it boils. Transfer them into a serving plate. Sprinkle with cilantro on top.

Apricot Smoothie

This smoothie makes 2 servings with 1 ½ cups each serving. This dish will take a total preparation time of 10 minutes. The following are the ingredients:

- 1 cup of canned apricots

- A cup of non-fat yogurt

- 6 ice cubes

- 3 tablespoons of sugar

Instructions:

Simply blend all the ingredients until it reaches the desired consistency. Every serving is composed of 6g protein, 3mg cholesterol, 0 fat, 202 calories, 74mg sodium, 49g carbohydrates, 2g fiber and 175 mg potassium.

Plum Spread for Diabetics

This homemade fruit spread contains less than ¼ the calories and 1/3 the carbohydrate of commercial plum spread. This method could also be done with peaches, strawberries and blackberries. This recipe will make 8 cups with a total preparation time of 60 minutes. The following are the ingredients:

- 15 cups of sliced plums

- ¾ cup of sugar

- 3 pieces of quartered (and washed) Granny Smith apples

- 2 tablespoons of lemon juice

- ¼ cup of grape fruit juice

- ¼ teaspoon of ginger or ground cinnamon

Instructions:

Start by placing the plate in a freezer. Meanwhile, combine grape juice, plums, and apple and lemon juice then put in a large Dutch oven. Boil over medium-high heat. Stir frequently. Afterwards, boil and cover. Stir occasionally for 20 minutes. Uncover. Boil gently. Stir occasionally until the fruit turns soft. Using a food mill, remove the skins and apple seeds. Return the processed fruit in the pot. Add cinnamon and sugar. Cook over medium-high heat. Stir frequently. Test whether the spoonful of jam will retain its shape after being dropped in a chilled plate. If it retains it shape, you may remove it from heat. Store the jam in a sealed container for up to two months.

This dish contains the following: 14 calories, 30 mg potassium and 4 g carbohydrates.

Mixed Veggies with Feta and Grapes

This dish will yield 8 servings of 1 ½ cups each. It will take 15 minutes to prepare. For the dressing, the following are the ingredients:

- ¼ cup of virgin olive oil

- ¼ teaspoon of salt

- Freshly ground pepper

- 2 tablespoons of red-wine vinegar

For the salad, the following are the ingredients:

- 5 ounces of salad greens

- 2 cups of seedless grapes (halved)

- ¾ cup of blue cheese

- 1 thinly-sliced radicchio

Instructions:

To prepare the dressing, simply combine all the dressing ingredients in a small bowl (together with salt and pepper) until the desired consistency is reached. To prepare the salad, toss the radicchio and greens in a big bowl. Drizzle the dressing on top. Divide the salad into 8 plates. Scatter the cheese and grapes equally on each plate. Serve immediately.

This dish has 133 calories, 10g fat, 9g carbohydrates, 1g fiber, 183mg potassium, 3g protein, 1g fiber, 239 mg sodium, and 13 mg cholesterol.

Tomato and Bread Salad

This recipe yields up to 6 servings of salad. It will take a total preparation time of 20 minutes. The following are the ingredients for this dish:

- 3 tablespoons of virgin olive oil

- 1 ½ pounds of seeded tomatoes

- 3 tablespoons of lemon juice

- 5 ounces of cubed whole-wheat country bread

- 1 clove of garlic

- ¼ cup of thinly sliced red onion

- ¼ teaspoon of salt

- 2 tablespoons of rinsed capers

- 5 cans of sardines

- Ground pepper

Instructions:

Simply whisk together pepper, garlic, oil, lemon juice, and salt in a big bowl. Add the bread, basil, tomatoes, onion and capers. Toss to combine. Let it sit for 5 minutes. Serve immediately.

This is composed of 168 calories, 107mg cholesterol, 3g of fiber, 22g protein, 657 sodium, 17g of fat, 19g carbohydrates, and 666 mg of potassium.

Green Beans and Nuts

This dish will yield 4 servings. It will take a total preparation time of 20 minutes. The following are the ingredients for this dish:

- 1 pound green beans

- ¼ teaspoon of salt

- 2 tablespoons of chopped hazelnuts

- 2 teaspoons of extra virgin olive oil

- Pepper

Instructions:

For 7 minutes, cook beans in a large pot of salt water. Drain well. Heat the oil in a medium-sized skillet over low heat. Add the nuts. Cook until golden. Add the beans. Season with pepper and salt.

This dish contains 104 calories, 9g carbohydrates, 5g fat, 4g fiber, 261 potassium, 152mg of sodium and 3g protein.

Pomegranate Seeds, Wild Rice and Barley Pilaf

This dish will yield up to 6 servings with ¾ cup each. It will take a total preparation time of 1 hour. The following are the ingredients for this recipe:

- 2 teaspoons of extra-virgin olive oil

- 3 cups of vegetable broth

- 1 finely chopped medium-sized onion

- 1 cup of pomegranate seeds

- 2 tablespoons of chopped parsley

- ½ cup of rinsed wild rice, ½ cup of barley

- 2 teaspoons of lemon zest (freshly grated)

Instructions:

Heat oil in a skillet over medium-high heat. Sauté onion until it softens. Drop in the barley and rice. Stir for a few seconds. Add the vegetable broth. Let it simmer. Reduce heat. Cover. Let it simmer for another 50 minutes. While waiting, toast the nuts in a dry skillet over medium-high heat. Stir constantly until the nuts turn light gold. Transfer the cooked nuts in a bowl to cool. Add the pomegranate seeds, parsley, and lemon zest in a bowl. Serve while hot.

This dish contains 209 calories, 3mg cholesterol, 7g protein 250mg potassium, 75 mg sodium, and 4g fiber.

Simple Roasted Chicken

This recipe yields up to 8 servings. This dish will take a total preparation and cooking time of 2 hours and 20 minutes. The following are the ingredients:

- 1 small onion (quartered and peeled)

- 5-pound chicken

- 3 cloves of garlic (quartered and peeled)

- 2 tablespoons of olive oil

- 4 sprigs of tarragon (preferably fresh)

- 1 teaspoon of kosher salt

- 4 sprigs of thyme (preferably fresh)

- ½ teaspoon of ground pepper

Instructions:

Pre-heat the oven until it reaches 380 °F. Place garlic, tarragon, onion and thyme inside the cavity of the chicken. Tie its legs together. Rub the chicken with pepper, salt and oil. Roast for 30 minutes.

This dish is composed of 180 calories, 300 mg sodium, 9g fat, 217 mg potassium, 64 mg cholesterol, and 1g carbohydrates.

Shrimp Bisque for Diabetics

This dish yields six servings with a cup each. It will take an hour and a half to prepare. The following are the ingredients for this dish:

- 12 ounces of shrimp

- ½ green bell pepper (finely chopped)

- 1 medium sized onion (finely chopped)

- 1/3 cup of scallions (finely chopped)

- 1 piece of peeled and sliced carrots

- 2 tablespoons of fresh parsley (finely chopped)

- 1 stalk celery

- ¼ cup of all-purpose flour

- 1/3 cup of white wine

- 2 cups of low-fat milk

- ½ teaspoon of black peppercorns

- ¼ cup of dry sherry

- 1 bay leaf

- 1 tablespoon of lemon juice

- 3 cups of water

- Pepper

- 1 tablespoon of olive oil

- Salt

- 4 ounces of mushrooms

- Hot sauce

Instructions:

Start by peeling and deveining the shrimp while reserving its shells. Cut the shrimp into one-inch pieces. Cover. Refrigerate. Combine the shells with half of the onion, celery, wine, peppercorns, bay leaf and carrots in a big saucepan. Add water. Let it simmer for half an hour. Strain well. Discard the solids. Keep only the liquids.

Afterwards, heat oil using the same pan over medium-high heat. Drop the remaining onion, bell pepper, scallions, parsley and mushrooms. Cook for 5 minutes. Sprinkle flour over the mixture while stirring constantly for 3 minutes. Add the milk and the shrimp stock slowly. Let it simmer for 5 minutes. Add the reserved shrimp and cook for 5 minutes. Add sherry, lemon juice and sour cream.

Make sure that the mixture does not come to a boil. Add salt, pepper and hot sauce according to taste.

This dish contains 163 calories, 92mg cholesterol, 13g protein, 1g fiber, 255 mg of potassium, 241 mg of sodium and 13g of protein.

Mangosteen Clinically Studied Formula

From extensive research, it seems a VERY high percentage of diseases like the diabetes can be preventable with proper nutrition

When it comes to the nutritional needs for you and your family, there's finally a single, ultra-premium, liquid formula that provides the vitamins, minerals and nutrients needed for optimal health.* Physician formulated and clinically studied formula, a health and wellness products superior to any other on the market with products for children and adults, for weight loss, cleansing, vitamins/minerals or just to maintain optimal health. After some research and trail I've become very happy with this companies specific products because not only do they have clinical studies done on the products that's shown to help with all type of diseases like joint pain, arthritis, reducing inflammation in body, lifting the T cell count and B cell count, boosting Immune System, lifting energy levels , diabetes and was even shown to help with some types of cancer and leukemia but they also have a money back guarantee if you're not satisfied. Here are some references on the clinical studies that are done; I hope this helps you on your journey to better health.

The journal of Medicinal Foods

https://www.vemma.com/pdf/JMF_clincalStudy.pdf

The Journal Of Agricultural And Food Chemistry

http://www.jbacademy.com/clinical-studies.pdf

To try their product go to:

http://www.Talalsobhi.vemma.com

Conclusion

Thank you again for downloading this book!

I hope this book was able to help you understand the diabetic diet. I also hope that you've realized just how easy it is to follow such a health-boosting eating regimen, especially since you could prepare and enjoy all sorts of tasty dishes.

The next step is to apply what you have learned!

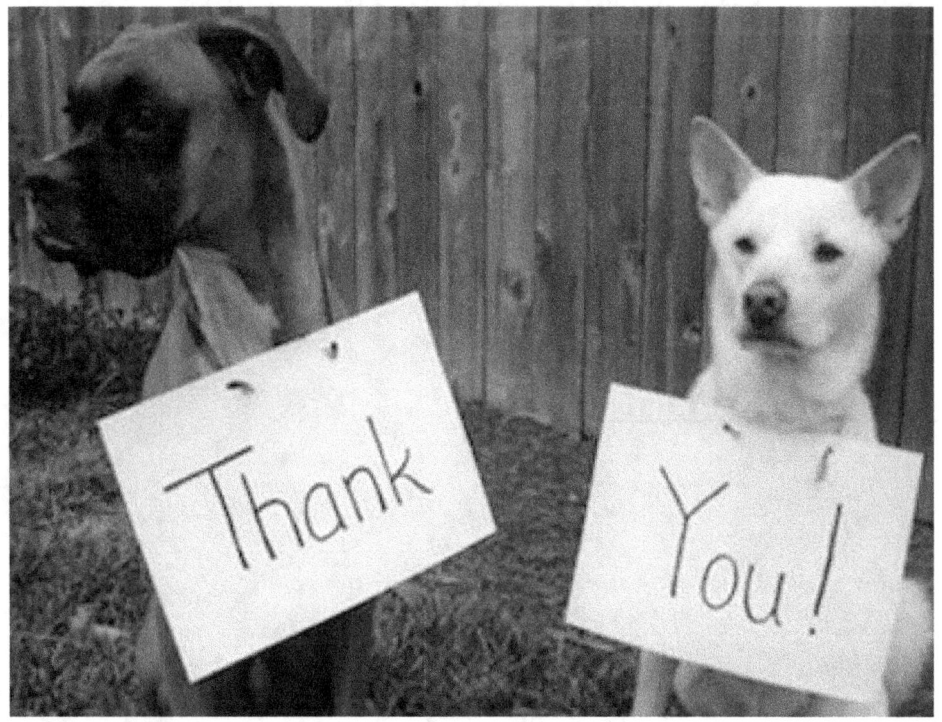

Finally, if you enjoyed this book, then I'd like to ask you for a favor, would you be kind enough to leave a review for this book on Amazon? It'd be greatly appreciated!

Thank you and good luck!

Talal.Sobhi

Check Out My Other Books

Below you'll find some of my other popular books that are popular on Amazon and Kindle as well. Simply click on the links below to check them out. Alternatively, you can visit my author page on Amazon to see other work done by me.

The True Jesus Speaks Out: The Biblical Secrets Revealed, Jesus Was Man Or Was Jesus God?

http://www.amazon.ca/gp/product/B00O349P2I?*Version*

The Ultimate Guide To Stress Free Parenting: How To become Stress Free Using Stress Free Management Skills.

http://www.amazon.ca/gp/product/B00NZI9XHU?

If the links do not work, for whatever reason, you can simply search for these titles on the Amazon website to find them.

Also add me to Facebook so we can chat:

http://www.facebook.com/talal.sobhey

This page is intentionally left blank

This page is intentionally left blank

This page is intentionally left blank

This page is intentionally left blank

This page is intentionally left blank

This page is intentionally left blank

This page is intentionally left blank